TABLE OF CONTENTS

INTRODUCTION

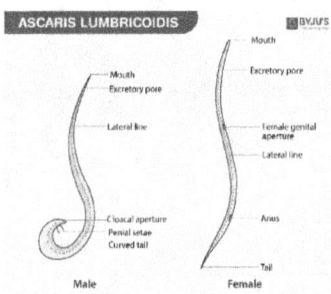

A nematode roundworm called Ascaris lumbricoides lives in the small intestine of people as parasites. These worms belong to the Ascarididae family, Secernentea class, and Oxyurida order. Pigs are a primary host of these worms. They are giant roundworms with three lips around their mouths that may grow to be 40 cm long. The small intestine is home to the Ascariasis infection that is brought on by Ascaris roundworms. Although this virus has no symptoms, children who are heavily infested may experience digestive problems, malnutrition, and development retardation. Around 807 million to 1.2 billion persons worldwide have ascariasis, a disease.

Stage 1: The Egg

The Egg Adult Ascaris worms are found inside the human small intestine. The female worm may reach a length of 35 cm and can produce 20,000 eggs, which are released into the environment along with the human faeces. Fertilised eggs are infectious and move on to the next stage of development whereas unfertilized eggs are swallowed but not infectious.

Stage 2; Larvae

Larvae are formed from fertilized eggs. After 18 days to several weeks, depending on the temperature, moisture, and soil type of the habitat, the larva then becomes infectious. The hatched larvae then penetrate the intestinal mucosa once the fertilised eggs have been consumed. They convey to other areas, including the lungs, from here. Then they go toward the throat so that the worms might be ingested and then sent back to the intestines to mature.

Stage 3: The Adult.

The larvae grow into adult worms once they enter the small intestine. The adult worm is now producing a lot of eggs. From the time infected eggs are consumed until female adult worms begin to lay their eggs, it takes around two to three months. A mature ascaris worm can live for one to two years.

Summary

Humans become infected with these worms when they ingest food or water tainted with Ascaris worm eggs. The two main hosts for Ascaris are humans and pigs. Dogs, monkeys, and other animals are also frequent hosts for Ascaris.

Animals known as parasites live off the body of another animal. In the human body, roundworms are among the most common parasites. In the human small intestine, there is a particular kind of roundworm called Ascaris.

Additionally, the roundworm species that causes this infection is Ascaris Lumbricoides. This illness is brought on by small intestine-dwelling larvae and adult worms, which grow there and reside there. The human body serves as a source of food as these worms develop. Additionally, mature worms may grow to a length of over 30 centimeters.

Soil contact is necessary for the minute ascariasis eggs to become infectious. Additionally, people may unintentionally consume any uncooked fruits or vegetables produced in contaminated soil, putting them in touch with the contaminated soil. In addition, failing to properly wash your hands before eating is another way to get this parasite.

Migration:

Ascaris lumbricoides' migration is the second stage of its life history. Within a person's small intestine, these eggs then develop into larvae. They then use the bloodstream or lymphatic system to get through the intestinal wall and enter the lungs. These larvae also spend about a week maturing in the lungs. After that, they enter the airway and are subsequently coughed up and ingested.

Maturation:

After returning to the colon, these parasites mature into either male or female worms. Female worms measure more than 40 centimetres (15 inches) in length and less than 6 millimetres (quarter inch) in diameter. However, male worms are smaller than female worms.

Reproductive:

The small intestine is where the reproduction process occurs. And female worms have a daily egg production capacity of about 200,000. By passing excrement, these eggs depart the human body. These fertilized eggs must also remain in the soil for at least 18 days before they become contagious.

The time it takes to effectively finish this procedure is also between two and three months. In addition, Ascaris can live for up to two years within a single person.

Acute Ascaris symptoms

When this parasite first appears, people are unable to recognize its symptoms. Patients may have symptoms like these when the infection in the small intestine begins,

- the inability to eat
- abdomen ache
- Vomiting
- stool showing signs of worms
- lose weight
- Diarrhoea
- Nausea
- inconsistent bowel movements

Furthermore, an individual may have the following symptoms if these parasites reach the lungs early on:

- Fever
- A coughing fit
- snotty mucus
- Anxiety in the chest
- Wheezing
- difficulty breathing

Identifying Ascaris

Stool samples are the main method used to determine whether the Ascaris suum life cycle is present in a patient. At the beginning of the infestation, this method might not be effective.

The quantity of eggs within a person may, however, always be determined with the use of imaging examinations. This can be accomplished through MRI, endoscopy, CT scans, ultrasounds, etc.

Ascaris treatment

To deal with this, anti-parasitic medications are typically administered. Surgery is the only treatment available in cases of serious illness,

Vaccination against Ascaris

Maintaining proper hygiene is the best defense against the Ascaris life cycle. You may avoid contracting this illness by washing your hands before eating and sanitising your produce.

If ignored for an extended period of time, the Ascaris life cycle may turn out to be a serious health problem. If not, it may be promptly treated properly and cured.

A kind of roundworm known as Ascaris Lumbricoides can cause an infection known as ascariasis when it affects the small intestines. Infections brought on by parasitic roundworms are quite frequent. Contaminated water or food can expose people to the virus. Usually, an infection does not create any symptoms, but if the infection or the number of worms rises, it may result in issues with the lungs or intestines.

Ascariasis causes

If someone consumes the eggs of Ascaris Lumbricoides, they may develop ascariasis. Eggs of the roundworm can be discovered in polluted water, raw food, or soil that has been exposed to human excrement. Children are more prone to get ascariasis, according to the WHO, if they play in contaminated dirt and put their hands in their mouths.

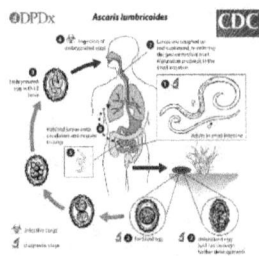

Life Cycle of an Ascaris

- In the lumen of the small intestine, adult worms can be found. About 20000 eggs are produced by a female and are excreted by her.
- The illness only spreads after 18 days to a few weeks in fertilized eggs; unfertilized eggs are not contagious.
- Warm, damp, shaded soil, for example, has an impact on the fertility of the eggs.
- In the small intestine, the larvae begin to hatch once the infectious eggs have been ingested.
- Later, the larvae go to the lungs through the circulation.
- Upon reaching adulthood, the larvae leave your lungs and go in the direction of your throat.
- Back in the intestines, the roundworms are once more ingested.

- Again mating in the intestines, the roundworms will produce additional eggs.
- Some eggs are expelled through the stool while others hatch and return to the lungs in this ongoing cycle.

Symptoms of Ascariasis

Roundworms in the Lungs: Signs and Symptoms
Fever
Uncomfortable chest
mucus with blood in it
Pulmonary aspiration
spitting up or coughing

Roundworms Symptoms

Roundworms in the Intestines: Signs and Symptoms
Nausea
Vomiting
diarrhoea or uncoordinated stools
intestine obstruction that causes vomiting or excruciating discomfort
worms that may be seen in the stool
reduced appetite
discomfort or pain in the abdomen

Ascariasis is identified

There are a few ways to identify acariasis:

1: Stool tests: Eggs and larvae can be found in the stools by using a microscope. Before the infection by at least 40 days, eggs do not show up in the stool.

2: Blood tests: Blood can be used to check for a rise in white blood cells, a sign that an infection may be present.

3: Abdominal X-rays Chest X-rays can show larvae in the lungs, whereas X-rays of the belly can show larvae in the abdomen.

4: Ultrasound—Ultrasound can make the liver or pancreatic larvae visible.

5: Using CT scans or MRIs, clinicians can find worms that are obstructing the ducts in the pancreas or the liver.

Treatment for ascariasis
Antiparasitic medications that kill the worms in two to three days are part of the treatment for the early stages of ascariasis. Surgery is needed to get rid of the worms and fix whatever harm they've done to the body when there is a severe infestation.

Protection against ascariasis

The prophylactic strategies used to prevent ascariasis include:

- observing excellent hygiene, which includes washing hands before and after using the restroom and before eating.
- Keep raw vegetables and food away from the sink.
- meal that is prepared, fresh, and healthful.

www.ingramcontent.com/pod-product-compliance
Lightning Source LLC
Chambersburg PA
CBHW080631220526
45467CB00011B/3460